Disclaimer

The information in this eBook reflects the opinions of the author and is not intended to replace medical or psychological advice, or any other professional advice. This EBook is not intended to diagnose or treat any psychological or medical conditions or disorders. If you are in need psychological or medical treatment, consult with a certified and licensed professional before determining whether the information in this book should be used.

Preface

There are various health problems which we are facing on a regular basis, there is a natural cure for all of these and is possible through te home remedies as well

In this book you will know about the benefits of foods vegetables and spices.

Cure at Home – Home and Natural care for Normal health Issues

Table of Contents

ACIDITY

Acidity is generally caused by an imbalance between the mechanism for secretion of acid in the stomach and the protective mechanism that ensures the stomach's safety. The stomach secretes acidic fluid that helps in digestion. But when the secretion of acid exceeds the normal level, it results in a situation termed as acidity.

Causes :- Inefficient digestive system Excessive intake of alcohol Empty stomach for a long time / skipping breakfast Eating foods rich in fats like chocolates Pregnancy Ageing Obesity Eating junk foods, oily and spicy foods Excessive exposure to sun and heat Aspirin and anti-inflammatory drugs Incompatibility of food Excess acid secretion Excessive smoking

- Acidity -

Causes :- Gastro duodenal (peptic) ulcer Hyper secretion of hydrochloric acid Reflux of gastric acid Negative emotions Weakness of the valves

Symptoms :- Chest pain Vomiting Coughing Heartburn Dyspepsia Belching Nausea Pain in the ears Inflammation in chest Respiratory problems Gastro-esophageal reflux Voice change and formation of ulcer in esophagus (tube connecting mouth and stomach) Pain during muscular contractions

- Acidity -

Symptoms :- Burning sensation or pain in the stomach after one to four hours of a meal Feel hungry frequently Constant pain in upper abdomen Bitter taste in mouth Loss of appetite

Foods to Avoid :- ☐ Alcohol ☐ Cabbage ☐ Fried food ☐ Non-veg diets ☐ Onion ☐ Pepper ☐ Pickles ☐ Radish ☐ Smoking ☐ Spicy, salty and acidic food ☐ Steroidal drugs

Foods to Eat :- ☐ Amaranth ☐ Apple ☐ Asparagus ☐ Banana ☐ Brazil nuts ☐ Fresh coconut ☐ Fresh peas ☐ Fresh vegetable juices ☐ Garlic ☐ Green beans

- Acidity -

Foods to Eat :- ☐ Buckwheat ☐ Carrots ☐ Celery ☐ Chestnuts ☐ Millet ☐ Parsley ☐ Sprouted Beans and seeds ☐ Watermelon

Remedies :-

◊ Drinking 3 tbsp white onion juice with 1 tbsp sugar and ½ cup curd helps to reduce acidity.

◊ Eating pineapple with sugar and pepper powder also reduces acidity.

◊ Consuming 1 tsp Indian gooseberry (amla) juice mixed with 11 gms of soaked and crushed black currant and ½ a tsp honey also helps to reduce acidity.

◊ Drinking chilled ¼ cup milk with ½ cup water relieves acidity.

◊ Consumption of chutney made with dry mangosteen, cardamom and sugar gives relief from acidity.

◊ Drinking ½ ltr of water mixed with ½ a tsp of sugar and juice of 1 lemon, ½ an hour before lunch, also reduces acidity.

◊ Eating a tsp of coriander powder mixed with ½ a tsp of sugar after meals also relieves you of acidity.

◊ Drinking carrot juice also works wonders in curing acidity.

◊ Mix powder of 4-5 pepper corns slowly roasted in ghee with 100 ml of milk and a little sugar and then drink it to reduce acidity.

- Acidity -

Remedies :-

◊ Consume 5-6 basil leaves with 1 cup curd or a glass of buttermilk to reduce acidity.

◊ Coriander powder and dry ginger powder mixed in equal quantities, and taking a teaspoon of this mixture reduces acidity.

~ ~ ~ ~ ~

ACNE

Acne is a skin disease caused by changes in the pilo-sebaceous units(the unit consists of the hair shaft, the hair follicle, the sebaceous gland which makes sebum, and the erector pili muscle which causes hair to stand up when it contracts) of a person. It usually strikes during adolescence but rarely continues till adulthood.

Commonly referred to as pimples, blemishes, spots and zits, acne lesions generally occur on the face, neck, chest, back, shoulders and upper arms. It may range from being mild and moderate to a severe form. While an increase in sex hormones, during puberty, is the leading cause for acne, there are other factors as well that add to its occurrence.

Causes :- Vitamin deficiency Over-activity of sebaceous glands Follicle fallout Bacterial infection Inflammation Sluggish liver Alcohol Hereditary factors Taking too much stress

- Acne -

Causes :- Misuse of drugs Hormonal imbalances Glucose intolerance Smoking Essential fatty acid deficiency Foods like pizza, chocolate, and fried items Cosmetics that are pore-clogging Pressure from helmets, chinstraps, collars, suspenders, etc Exposure to industrial products, like cutting oils Environmental irritants, such as polluted air and high humidity Squeezing or picking at blemishes Hard scrubbing of the skin Change of hormonal levels in women, mainly before, during and after menses Congested colon and constipation Food allergies and food sensitivities, especially to milk Medications that contain bromides, iodides or steroids

The contraceptive pill can improve acne for some, but worsen for others, depending on the balance of estrogen and progesterone in the brand of the pill.

- Acne -

Symptoms:- Greasy skin Blackheads Cysts Scars Nodules Papules Whiteheads Red or yellow spots (pustules) Deep, inflamed lesions Pimples on the face and upper torso

Foods to Avoid :- ☐ Alcohol ☐ Butter ☐ Cheese ☐ Chips ☐ Coffee ☐ Cookies ☐ Cream ☐ Deep fried food ☐ Pasta ☐ Pork ☐ Processed grains ☐ Red meat ☐ Salami ☐ Sausage ☐ Soya sauce ☐ Sugary and carbonated

- Acne -

Foods to Avoid :- ☐ Ham ☐ Ice cream ☐ Liver drinks ☐ Tea ☐ Vinegar ☐ White breads

Foods to Eat :- ☐ Apricots fresh or dried ☐ Avocado ☐ Cantaloupe melon ☐ Carrots ☐ Cherries ☐ Chicken ☐ Egg ☐ Flaxseed ☐ Grapefruit ☐ Green tea ☐ Guava ☐ Lean red meat ☐ Mango ☐ Multi-Grain Breads ☐ Oatmeal ☐ Oranges ☐ Plantain ☐ Pomegranate ☐ Salmon ☐ Skim or 1% milk ☐ Walnut ☐ Watermelon

Remedies :-

◊ Mix equal quantities of glycerin, rose water and lime juice and store it in a bottle. Massage with this liquid daily on all the

- Acne -

Remedies :-

exposed parts of skin to get a glow in a very short time.

◊ To get a glow on the skin, mix a little curd with radish juice and massage with this mixture daily.

◊ To get a soft and glowing skin, squeeze the juice of a whole lime in a bucketful of warm or cold water and then bathe with it.

◊ To cure any kind of old skin diseases apply bitter gourd juice on the skin, let it dry for few minutes and then take a bath.

◊ To bring a glow, apply sesame seed oil daily.

◊ To get a wrinkle free skin, apply cucumber juice, let it dry and then wash it off.

◊ To get a blemishes free skin, dry a few orange peel, make a powder and make a paste by mixing little rose water, apply this on face, let it dry, and then wash it off with cold water.

◊ In cases where there are cracks in legs and hands or even prickly heat, mix 1 portion of lemon juice with 3 parts of sesame oil or coconut oil and apply it to the affected parts.

◊ To get a fairer and glowing skin, mix little water and ghee with gram flour and apply during bath, instead of soap.

◊ In cases of scars left over after burns, apply coconut oil regularly over the scars.

◊ To cure many skin diseases like irritation, boils and scars mix 20-22 gms honey with cold water and drink it daily in empty stomach.

- Acne -

Remedies :-

◊ To get a beautiful and glowing skin, mix water with which rice has been washed; with turmeric powder, apply just before bathing.

◊ Apply malai (fresh cream) on the face half an hour before bathing, scrub it off with hands on drying and then wash it off to get a beautiful and glowing skin.

◊ To make skin soft, scrub raw potato peel over the skin.

◊ To unclog the pores and to get a glowing skin, scrub used lime peel for few minutes on the skin.

◊ To get a fair and beautiful skin mix amla (Indian gooseberry) powder with turmeric powder and milk and apply it and wash it after drying. Repeat this process daily for a few months.

◊ Boil 1 litre of water till it reduces to half, and then mix equal quantities of glycerin and lime juice, mix thoroughly and store it in a bottle. Wash your face with this liquid 2-3 times in a day. It keeps your skin cool in the summer and prevents it from drying in winter.

~ ~ ~ ~ ~

ANAEMIA

Anaemia is a decrease in the normal number of red blood cells (RBCs) or less than the normal quantity of haemoglobin in the blood. However, it can include decreased oxygen-binding ability of each haemoglobin molecule due to deformity or lack of numerical development as in some other types of haemoglobin deficiency.

Anaemia is the most common disorder of the blood. There are several kinds of Anaemia, produced by a variety of underlying causes. Anaemia can be classified in a variety of ways. The three main classes of Anaemia include excessive blood loss, excessive blood cell destruction and deficient red blood cell production.

Causes :- Blood loss Decreased or faulty red blood cell production Destruction of red blood cells Hereditary disorders Poor absorption of iron, low stomach acid and a vegan diet, as B12 is mainly found in animal foods such as fish, meat and eggs

- Anaemia -

Symptoms :- Lack of energy Dizziness Indigestion Poor bodily repair Edema Constipation Loss of appetite Depression Poor hair condition Cold hands and feet Breathlessness on exertion Reduced muscular strength Increased susceptibility to infections Yellow tinge to the skin A red, beefy and sore tongue Bleeding under the skin Weak heartbeat and numb feet Brittle and ridged finger nails

- Anaemia -

Foods to Avoid :- ☐ Alcohol ☐ Beer ☐ Bran ☐ Chocolate ☐ Ice cream ☐ Rhubarb ☐ Smoking ☐ Soft drinks ☐ Sorrel (a herb) ☐ Tea and coffee

Foods to Eat :- ☐ Almonds ☐ Apples ☐ Asparagus ☐ Baked beans ☐ Bananas ☐ Beef liver ☐ Black-eyed peas ☐ Brazil nuts ☐ Broccoli ☐ Brussels sprouts ☐ Butter beans ☐ Cantaloupe ☐ Carrots ☐ Haricot beans ☐ Iron-fortified cereals ☐ Kidney beans ☐ Lean, red meat ☐ Lemons ☐ Lentils ☐ Oatmeal ☐ Oranges ☐ Oysters ☐ Peas ☐ Pinto beans ☐ Plums ☐ Poultry

- Anaemia -

Foods to Eat :- ☐ Cashew nuts ☐ Chickpeas ☐ Collard greens ☐ Dried fruit ☐ Figs ☐ Fish ☐ Ginger ☐ Grapes ☐ Green, leafy vegetables ☐ Raisins ☐ Romaine lettuce ☐ Sesame seeds ☐ Spinach ☐ Tomatoes ☐ Walnuts ☐ Wheat germ ☐ Whole grain cereals

Remedies :-

◊ Avoid drinking tea and coffee immediately after meals as the tannin present in these interferes in the absorption of iron from food.

◊ Take freshly prepared apple juice just before going to bed or half an hour before a meal. For proper absorption of the juice, stomach should be relatively empty and do not take anything for at least next 30 minutes.

◊ Beetroot juice is an excellent remedy for Anaemia. Apple may also be added to the juice.

◊ Mix 1 tbsp amla juice with a ripe mashed banana and eat 2-3 times a day.

- Anaemia -

Remedies :-

◊ Have a ripe banana with 1 tbsp of honey, 1-2 times a day.

◊ Soak 10-12 currants in water overnight. Remove seeds and eat them. Have this for 2-4 weeks.

◊ Try to have at least 100 gms of green leafy vegetable like spinach, lettuce, celery, fenugreek everyday, raw or cooked.

~ ~ ~ ~ ~

ANOREXIA NERVOSA

Anorexia nervosa is characterized by an irrational fear of becoming fat coupled with a relentless pursuit of thinness. People with anorexia go to extremes to reach and maintain a dangerously low body weight. But no matter how much weight is lost, no matter how emaciated they become, it's never enough. The more the scale dips, the more obsessed they become with food, dieting, and weight loss.

The key features of anorexia nervosa are:

• Refusal to sustain a minimally normal body weight.

• Intense fear of gaining weight, despite being underweight.

• Distorted view of one's body or weight, or denial of the dangers of one's low weight.

Causes :- Dissatisfaction with own body Dieting Low self-esteem Obsession with perfectionism Childhood sexual abuse Family history of eating disorders Genetics

- Anorexia Nervosa -

Causes :- Individual personality traits Family environment Participation in activities like ballet, gymnastics etc

Symptoms :- Dieting despite being thin Obsession with calories, fat grams, and nutrition Pretending to eat or lying about eating Preoccupation with food Strange or secretive food rituals Loss of menstrual periods Lack of energy and weakness Feeling cold all the time Dry, yellowish skin Constipation and abdominal pain Infertility Stunted growth Osteoporosis Heart problems Kidney failure Depression

- Anorexia Nervosa -

Symptoms :- Dramatic weight loss Feeling fat, despite being underweight Fixation with body image Harshly critical of own appearance Denies being too thin Using diet pills, laxatives, or diuretics Throwing up after eating Compulsive exercising Restlessness and insomnia Dizziness, fainting, and headaches Growth of fine hair all over the body and face Severe mood swings Thoughts of suicide Tooth and gum decay

Foods to Avoid :- ☐ Alcohol ☐ Caffeine ☐ Tobacco ☐ Refined sugars, such as candies ☐ Soft drinks

- Anorexia Nervosa -

Foods to Eat :- ☐ Avocados ☐ Bananas ☐ Brown rice ☐ Herring ☐ High carbohydrate foods ☐ High fat foods ☐ High protein foods ☐ Legumes ☐ Miso soup ☐ Nut butters ☐ Oat cakes ☐ Pulses ☐ Pumpkin seeds ☐ Quinoa ☐ Sesame seeds ☐ Smoothies ☐ Sunflower seeds ☐ Watercress ☐ Wheat germ

Remedies :-

◊ Eating crushed ginger a few minutes before meals will increase appetite.

◊ Drinking mint juice with rock salt also helps to increase hunger.

◊ Mixing rock salt, ½ a tsp carom seeds powder (ajwain powder) and lime juice (sweet) does increase hunger.

◊ To increase appetite and hunger, mix lime juice and honey with lukewarm water and drink it daily.

◊ Chewing ½ a tsp of ajwain seeds twice daily also increases appetite.

◊ Eating a tsp of mustard powder with water also helps.

- Anorexia Nervosa -

Remedies :-

◊ Eating pineapple with pepper powder and rock salt also helps a lot.

◊ Sprinkle a little rock salt over ½ a lime and the suck the juice a little before meals.

◊ Taking ¼ tsp asafoetida with ½ tsp ghee also increases appetite.

◊ Mix onion juice with asafoetida and salt and then drink it.

◊ Let the finely chopped garlic crackle in oil and then eat it; or make a paste of it and have it with your meals.

◊ Boil 4-5 dry mangosteen in 1 cup water and drink this water with ghee.

~ ~ ~ ~ ~

ARTHRITIS

The literal meaning of arthritis is "joint inflammation" and it can affect joints in any part of the body. When you have arthritis, damage is caused to a lesser or greater degree to the joints and mostly occurs in the hands, arms and legs. The inflammation in one or more of the joints results in pain, swelling and limited movement.

Causes :- Broken bone Infection in the area (usually caused by either bacteria or viruses) An autoimmune disease (this is where the body attacks itself because the immune system perceives a certain body part to be foreign) General wear and tear of joints (possibly from old age, over exercise etc.) Injury (leading to osteoarthritis) Metabolic abnormalities (such as gout and pseudo gout) Hereditary factors Infections Certain unclear reasons (such as rheumatoid arthritis)

- Ar thri t i s -

Causes :- Hormonal imbalance Emotional stress Structural changes in the particular cartilage of any joint Physical exertion Severe fright Shock Obesity Ageing Previous physical injuries

Occupational hazards, such as those experienced by assembly line workers and heavy construction High-level sports

Symptoms :- Anaemia Colitis Constipation Weak digestion Intermittent fever Loss of appetite Fever

- Ar thri t i s -

Symptoms :- Overeating Weight loss Fatigue Feeling unwell Joint pain and swelling Stiffness particularly in the mornings Abnormalities of organs such as the lungs, heart, or kidneys A feeling of warmth around a joint Redness of skin around an affected joint Stiffness in the joints Deformed hands and feet Inflammation of muscles, ligaments and cartilage Painful movement of the joints, especially in cold, windy and damp weather Very little physical activity Blotchy rash on the arms and legs Inability to move the joints easily Tenderness of the inflamed joint Gland swelling (lymph node)

- Ar thri t i s -

Foods to Avoid :- ☐ Beans ☐ Biscuits ☐ Cakes ☐ Chocolate ☐ Coffee ☐ Dairy products ☐ Fried foods ☐ Meat ☐ Pastry ☐ Preservatives and additives ☐ Tea ☐ Tomatoes

Foods to Eat :- ☐ Almonds ☐ Apples ☐ Asparagus ☐ Avocado ☐ Banana ☐ Beetroot ☐ Blueberries ☐ Brazil nuts ☐ Broccoli ☐ Button mushrooms ☐ Cantaloupe ☐ Carrots ☐ Cauliflower ☐ Mango ☐ Onion ☐ Oranges ☐ Papaya ☐ Peach ☐ Peas ☐ Peppers ☐ Pineapple ☐ Plums ☐ Pumpkin seeds ☐ Sardines ☐ Sockeye salmon ☐ Spinach

- Ar thri t i s -

Foods to Eat :- ☐ Celery ☐ Cherries ☐ Collards ☐ Ginger ☐ Grapefruit ☐ Grapes ☐ Green vegetables ☐ Herring ☐ Kiwi Fruit ☐ Linseeds ☐ Squash ☐ Strawberries ☐ Sunflower seeds ☐ Sweet corn ☐ Sweet potato ☐ Turmeric ☐ Walnuts ☐ Whole or cracked grains ☐ Winter squashes

Remedies :-

◊ A gentle massage with olive oil will give a lot of relief.

◊ Take equal amounts of water and freshly extracted potato juice and drink it daily.

◊ Rub the aching joints with hot vinegar just before going to bed.

◊ Take 10 gms of camphor and put it in a glass bottle filled with 100 gms of mustard oil. Keep this bottle in the sun till the camphor dissolves. Apply this oil in the joints daily.

◊ A teaspoon of black sesame seeds, soaked in a quarter cup of water and kept overnight, has been found to be effective in preventing frequent joint pains. The water in which the seeds

- Ar thri t i s -

Remedies :-

are soaked should also be taken along with the seeds first thing in the morning.

◊ Drinking water kept overnight in a copper container accumulates traces of copper, which is said to strengthen the muscular system. A copper ring or bracelet is worn for the same reason.

◊ Garlic is another effective remedy for arthritis. Garlic may be taken raw or cooked according to individual preference.

◊ Bananas, being a rich source of vitamin B6, have proved useful in the treatment of arthritis. A diet of only bananas for three or four days is advised in treating this condition. The patient may eat eight or nine bananas daily during this period and nothing else.

◊ A green gram soup should be prepared by mixing a tablespoon of green gram in a cup of water, with two crushed garlic cloves. It should be taken twice a day.

◊ Add one tablespoon of cod liver oil to the juice of one orange, whip and drink before going to bed.

~ ~ ~ ~ ~

WONDER FOODS

- Spices / Herbs -

Wonder Food : Spices

- Spices / Herbs -

ANISEED / FENNEL

For centuries, people wanting to lose weight and stay young ate fennel seeds. However, fennel seeds are most effective as a digestive agent – settling the stomach, relieving colic and wind, and easing indigestion and heartburn. It can also boost your appetite. It is also an antispasmodic and diuretic. It can also act as an antioxidant. It will also help to increase milk production in lactating mothers.

Tea made with a few fresh sprigs of fennel or a level teaspoon of seeds will relieve indigestion. An infusion of the seeds is an excellent carminative, especially for babies.

Fennel is an effective treatment for respiratory congestion and is a common ingredient in cough remedies. An essential oil is often extracted from the seed for medicinal use, though it should not be given to pregnant women.

Recipe : Braised Fennel With Cheese Nutritional Value (approx.)

Energy

Protein

Carbohydrate

Fat

1488

50 g

213 g

67 g

Nutritional Value (100 gms) Calorie 345 Protein 15.8 g Carbohydrate 52.29 g Fat 14.87 g Fiber 39.8 g

- Spices / Herbs -

Ingredients :- □ Butter – 50 g □ Baby fennel bulbs – 12 □ Water – 150 ml □ Juice of 1 lemon □ Salt and Pepper – to taste □ Balsamic vinegar – 1 tbsp □ Cheese, grated – 3-4 tbsp

Method :- ◊ Melt butter in a large pan. When it stops foaming, add trimmed and halved fennel bulbs lengthways. ◊ Sauté gently for 2 minutes on each side until light golden. ◊ Add water and lemon juice. Add salt and pepper, bring to boil, cover and simmer for 20 minutes or until the fennel is tender. ◊ Add vinegar and increase the heat to reduce the liquid by half. ◊ Remove the pan from the heat. Add the cheese. Allow the cheese to melt. ◊ Serve hot.

Recipe : Aniseed Sherbat Nutritional Value (approx.)

Energy

Protein

Carbohydrate

Fat

885

41 g

144 g

36 g

- Spices / Herbs -

Ingredients :- □ Aniseed powder – 1 cup □ Sugar Powder – ¾ cup ◻ Cardamom powder – of 4-5

Method :- ◊ Mix all the ingredients together and sieve and store it in the refrigerator. ◊ Whenever required, add 2-3 tsp of the powder to 1 glass of cold water and serve. ◊ It is a great coolant in the hot summer. ◊ Drinking it everyday just before going out in the sun will prevent you from getting affected by the warm winds.

~ ~ ~ ~ ~

- Spices / Herbs -

ASAFOETIDA

Asafoetida is dirty yellow in color with a pungent smell.

It is extensively used in the treatment of nervous disorders of children. There is an old European belief that a small piece of this gum, hung around a child's neck, would protect it from many diseases, especially germs which are sensitive to its particular odor.

Asafoetida is known for its medicinal properties since ages and has been in use as a medicine in India, in antispasmodic and anti-flatulent mixtures.

It is useful in respiratory conditions like whooping cough, upper respiratory tract infections where congestion is a problem, asthmatic attacks and bronchitis. One ayurvedic school of thought has recommended asafoetida in classical hysteric attacks. It is also an effective remedy for toothache. In general it helps in preventing dental caries or at least in relieving pain due to caries.

Asafoetida is considered useful in the treatment of several problems concerning women such as sterility, unwanted abortion, pre-mature labor, unusually painful, difficult and excessive menstruation and leucorrhoea. It is also beneficial in the treatment of impotency.

Asafoetida is known to Indian society from ages and is widely used as flavouring agent in Indian recipes. It is considered as a safe home made remedy for digestive disturbances until one sees the doctor. In short, Nutritional Value (100 gms) Calorie 297 Protein 4.0 g Carbohydrate 67.8 g Fat 1.1 g Fiber 4.1 g

- Spices / Herbs -

asafoetida is a medicinal gum of the plant used in stomach disorders like nausea, anorexia and flatulence. Taken internally or applied externally it helps in relieving distention of abdomen due to improper digestion or gases.

Recipe : Moong Dal Hing Kachori Nutritional Value (approx.)

Energy

Protein

Carbohydrate

Fat

1060

55 g

215 g

15 g

Ingredients :- ☐ Moong Dal (cooked) – 1 cup For Filling: ☐ Green chilies (minced) - 3 ☐ Mint leaves – 4-5 ☐ Coriander leaves chopped finely – 2 tbsp ☐ Curry leaves – 1 sprig ☐ Salt - to taste ☐ Shredded Ginger – 1 tsp ☐ Ghee – 2 tbsp ☐ Asafoetida – 1 tsp ☐ Cumin Seeds – ½ tsp ☐ Aniseeds – ¼ tsp ☐ Mango powder – ½ tsp ☐ Turmeric powder - ½ tsp ☐ Garam Masala - 1 tsp ☐ Chili Powder - 1 tsp For the Covering (dough): ☐ Refined Flour – 1 ½ cup ☐ Ghee – 2 tbsp ☐ Salt - to taste ☐ Oil/Ghee - for deep frying

- Spices / Herbs -

Method :- ◊ Knead a soft pliable dough and set aside. ◊ Take half the quantity of cooked dal and mash it and keep half of the dal aside. ◊ Melt the ghee and fry the green chilies, mint, coriander leaves, and curry leaves, then add the cumin seeds and aniseeds and fry till it splutters. ◊ Add the mashed dal, and the whole dal, garam masala, mango powder, turmeric powder, chili powder, salt and fry on low heat till dry. ◊ Remove and set aside to let it cool. ◊ In the meantime heat up the oil/ghee in a wok for frying. ◊ While it is getting hot, make small puris, putting a tbsp of the dal mixture in the center and gathering the ends of the circle and firmly pressing the gathering, and then slightly flatten with palm and deep fry till golden brown. ◊ Serve with chutney or sauce.

~ ~ ~ ~ ~

- Spices / Herbs -

BASIL

The herb Basil is used in cooking universally, and also for medicinal purposes. It's a great herb and everyone should consider using it in their diet.

Jews believe (an enduring belief) that eating basil provides strength when fasting. It is used as tonic for the skin, a treatment for all kinds of colds, bronchitis, and coughs. It is used to treat gas attacks, flu, gout, muscle aches, rheumatism, insect bites, and sinusitis. An infusion of the green herb in boiling water is good for all obstructions of the internal organs, arrests vomiting and nausea. It is often used as an insect repellent.

In West Africa it is used to reduce fevers and the Japanese use it as a cold remedy. As basil is both aromatic and carminative, it is used for mild nervous disorders and even for the alleviation of fibromyalgia(wandering body pains). It is said, the dried leaves used as a snuff, can cure nervous headaches. In traditional Ayurvedic medicine, a variety of Indian basil has been used to treat many common ailments, and naturopathic physicians may prescribe it in the treatment of diabetes, respiratory disorders, impotence, allergies and infertility.

Basil is also known to have extremely powerful antioxidant properties, especially when it is used in the form of an extract or oil. The natural Nutritional Value (100 gms) Calorie 23 Protein 3.15 g Carbohydrate 2.65 g Fat 0.64 g Fiber 1.6 g antioxidants found in basil can protect the body against damage from free radicals, thereby preventing cellular ageing, common skin ailments, and even most forms of cancer. Antioxidants are an important part of maintaining a healthy diet and lifestyle, and basil may be a safe and effective source of these potent, life-giving compounds.

Basil is not only a herb that does you good, it also tastes good, so make sure you get plenty in your diet.

Recipe : Tulsi Ka Kadha Nutritional Value (approx.)

Energy

Protein

Carbohydrate

Fat

35

2 g

11 g

1 g

Ingredients :- ☐ Water – 1 glass ☐ Basil Leaves – 10-12 pieces ☐ Ginger, grated – ½ inch ☐ Cinnamon – 1 inch ☐ Clove -2 ☐ Cardamom, slightly crushed – 2 ☐ Bay leaf – 1 ☐ Honey or Jaggery – to taste

Spices / Herbs -

Method :- ◊ Mix all the ingredients together and boil till the mixture reduces to half. ◊ Strain and drink it warm.

~ ~ ~ ~ ~

CARDAMOM / ELAICHI

Cardamom too, is used for cooking as well as for medicinal purposes. It is used in a variety of dishes and is used to treat the teeth and gums just like clove is used. However, it is also used to treat throat problems, pulmonary tuberculosis and inflammation of eyelids, lung congestion and digestive disorders. It is also used to develop an antidote for venom of snakes and scorpions.

In traditional medicine, it has been used for treating constipation, dysentery, stomach aches and other types of digestive problems. It will serve as an excellent diuretic for the treatment of gonorrhea, cystitis, nephritis, burning micturation or urination and scanty urination. This can be used as a remedy for the treatment of depression. The herb is useful in sexual dysfunctions like impotency and premature ejaculation. But excessive use of cardamom at times may lead to impotency.

Gargling with an infusion of cardamom and cinnamon cures pharyngitis, sore-throat, relaxes uvula, or the fleshy conical portion at the back of the tongue, and hoarseness during the infective stage of influenza. Indeed, cardamom is a herb that is widely used in foods as well as it is a remedy for a number of stomach and respiratory tract ailments.

Cardamom is the only versatile herb that gives a cooling effect if used in any preparation in summer and gives a warm effect in winter.

Nutritional Value (100 gms) Calorie 311 Protein 10.76 g Carbohydrate 68.47 g Fat 6.7 g Fiber 28 g

- Spices / Herbs -

Recipe : Elaichi Tea Nutritional Value (approx.)

Energy

Protein

Carbohydrate

Fat

104

8 g

13 g

2 g

Ingredients :- ☐ Milk – 1 cup ☐ Water – 1 cup ☐ Sugar – to taste ☐ Tea leaves – as desired ☐ Cardamom, slightly crushed – 2-3

Method :- ◊ Mix all the ingredients together. ◊ Boil for 2-3 minutes till you get the desired color. ◊ Strain and serve hot.

~ ~ ~ ~ ~

- Fruits -

Wonder Food : Fruits

- Fruits -

APPLE

It was said long ago, 'to eat an apple before going to bed will make the doctor beg his bread'. The modern version of this ancient saying, 'an apple a day keeps the doctor away', sums up the healthful and nourishing qualities of apples. Apples are invaluable for the maintenance of good health and in the treatment of many ailments.

Apples detoxify the body and have an antiviral property. Apples are known to remove weakness and add vigour and vitality. It is, therefore, often given to patients to help them recover fast from their illness. It lowers cholesterol and risk of cancer. Has mild antibacterial, anti-viral, anti-inflammatory estrogenic activity. High in fiber, helps avoid constipation, suppresses appetite. Juice can cause diarrhea in children.

The cancer fighting qualities contained in a fresh, unpeeled apple are impressive. There are numerous studies whose findings are promising to anyone seeking to prevent or treat cancer.

Lung cancer was not the only form of cancer worked on by apples. Many of the studies previously cited proved apple's value with other forms of cancer as well. Among these are; prostate cancer, colon cancer, breast cancer and leukemia. A list of known biological activities associated with apples include: anticancer, antileukemic, antimutagenic, antimetastic, Nutritional Value (100 gms) Calorie 354 Protein 7.83 g Carbohydrate 64.93 g Fat 9.88 g Fiber 21.1 g

- Fruits -

antineoplastic (stomach), antiproliferant and antitumor and acts specifically on the skin, pancreas, stomach, breast and bladder.

In addition to important cancer fighting constituents, apples aid the digestive system and related diseases. First of all, apples fight obesity. The fiber in the form of pectin is just one factor that affects weight. The pectin has an amphoteric action. This means it is either laxative or antidiarrheal, according to the body's needs.

Pectin can interfere with the body's ability to absorb dietary fats. Obesity is a huge factor in Type II diabetes. Blood sugar is also a factor. Pectin aids in the reduction of blood sugar. So, in addition to apple's antiobesity, nutritive and digestive qualities, is revealed its antidiabetic action.

The malic acid in an apple is beneficial for the bowels, liver and brain. Apples are cleaners. Among some of the reported actions are benefits for those exposed to radiation. It has been reported that apples are beneficial in binding radioactive residues and helping to excrete them from the body. Apples can also help remove toxic metals like lead from the body.

Maybe one of the most important cleaning actions provided by apples has to do with cholesterol. The pectin, as well as other constituents, plays a role in reducing bad cholesterol in the body. This is good news for blood vessels and the heart. Because apple is also a hematic, it can build blood as well as cleanse it.

A reduced risk of cardiovascular disease has been associated with apple consumption. This same study showed apple's constituents to have an effect on cerebrovascular health. The apple provides antioxidants for the body. Oxidative damage on cells by free radicals contributes to age

- Fruits -

related brain disorders. Alzheimer's and senility are examples. Apples have been cited as antialzheimerian.

The apple also contains qualities that help prevent the eye and nerve damage associated with diabetes.

Most of the apples medicinal qualities treat chronic illness. 'An apple a day' is an important adage to follow in order to enjoy its effects in these areas. There are many more benefits inherent in an apple. One source cites; Antianaemic, antibacterial, anti-inflammatory, antimenopauseal, antiCrohn's, antiedemic, anti PMS, antiseptic, antiyeast, antiviral, capillary protective, hepatoprotective, diuretic, fungicide, nematicide (round worms), and neuroprotective are a few not mentioned before. Still other sources assign tonic, astringent, disinfectant, cardiac stimulant and cephalic.

Recipe : Apple Streusel Pie Nutritional Value (approx.)

Energy

Protein

Carbohydrate

Fat

3797

46 g

640 g

124 g

Ingredients :- ☐ Baking or pie apples - 8 ☐ Sugar – 1 cup ☐ Cinnamon – 1 tsp ☐ Pie crust - 1 deep-dish ☐ Flour – ¾ cup For the pie crust ☐ Whole wheat flour – 1 cup, mixed with white flour – ½ cup ☐ Salt - ½ tsp

- Fruits -

Ingredients :- ☐ Margarine – ½ cup ☐ Butter - ½ -cup ☐ Cold milk or water -5 tbsp

Method :- Method for Pie Crust ◊ Sift flours and salt together; use all the bran that is sifted. ◊ Crumb the butter into the flour; rub in until it becomes crumbly. ◊ Add liquid a spoonful at a time, mixing and pressing together until dough is moist enough to hold together. ◊ This makes a 2-crust pie. ◊ Halve the quantity if base of pie only is required. Method for the pie: ◊ Pre-heat the oven to 180°C / 350°F. ◊ Peel and slice the apples and place in a large bowl. ◊ In a small bowl, mix ½ cup of the sugar and cinnamon. Add to the apples until they are coated. ◊ Put the apples in the pie crust. ◊ Mix the remaining ½ cup sugar, the flour and margarine until

- Fruits -

Method :- crumbly. Add a small amount of flour if necessary until small crumbs form. ◊ Sprinkle the crumbs over the pie, covering completely. ◊ Garnish with apple slices. ◊ Bake for 40 minutes until slightly browned.

~ ~ ~ ~ ~

- Fruits -

APRICOT

Throughout the centuries, the fruit, kernels, oil and flowers of the apricot have been used in medicine. In China, a famous medicine known as 'Apricot Gold' was made from the kernels of trees which grew in certain areas. This medicine was reputed for its powers to prolong life. The Chinese also believed that apricots reacted sympathetically to women's ailments. The apricot flowers, therefore, formed a common ingredient in their cosmetics.

The kernel, which yields oil similar to that of the almond, has been widely used for their sedative, antispasmodic (which gives relief to strained muscles) and demulcent or soothing properties. They are useful in the healing of wounds, in expelling worms and as a general tonic.

The fruit is highly valued as a gentle laxative and is beneficial in the treatment of constipation. Patients suffering from chronic constipation can greatly benefit by the regular use of apricots.

Apricots have an alkaline reaction in the system. They aid digestion, if consumed before a meal. Marmalade, made from organically grown fruit, is also valuable in the treatment of nervous indigestion.

The apricot is an excellent food remedy for anaemia on account of its high content of iron. The small but essential amount of copper in the fruit makes iron available to the body. Liberal use of apricots could also increase the production of haemoglobin in our body. Nutritional Value (100 gms) Calorie 48 Protein 1.4 g Carbohydrate 11.12 g Fat 0.39 g Fiber 2 g

- Fruits -

Fresh juice of apricots, mixed with glucose or honey, is a very cooling drink during fevers. It quenches thirst and eliminates the waste products from the body. It tones up the eyes, stomach, liver, heart and nerves by supplying vitamins and minerals. Fresh juice of apricot leaves is useful for treating skin diseases. It can be applied with beneficial results in scabies, eczema, sun-burn and itching of the skin due to cold exposure.

Apricot seeds, because of their remarkably high content of amygdalin, are a source of vitamin B17 and utilized in alternative medicine for cancer therapy. It has to be underlined, however, that the seeds must be baked prior to direct consumption, since apricot kernels can be poisonous if ingested raw in large quantities.

It prevents plaque-deposits from building up in the arteries, helps to strengthen our immune system and is beneficial to eyes, skin, hair, gums and various glands.

Apricot and apricot products help to maintain body fluid balance by normalizing blood pressure and heart function. Boron, which apricots are also rich in, has lately been identified as one of the main factors for the prevention of osteoporosis, by helping post-menopausal women retain their estrogen levels.

The almost endless list of the amazing nutritional and medicinal properties of apricot fruits and kernels can go on and on. It is not surprising that dried apricots being compact, balanced and rich in minerals, macro and microelements were the NASA's number one choice as astronauts' provision. It is a warming, bitter-sweet herb which helps in controlling coughing. The laetrile contained in the pip is used in cancer

- Fruits -

therapy. It must however be noted that excessive amounts of the pip can be toxic.

Safety precautions and warnings - Excessive intake of the amygdalin contained in apricots can cause nervous system depression and respiratory failure. Eating the unripe fruit can cause gastric disorder.

Recipe : Pan-Fried Apricots With Gingered Mascarpone Nutritional Value (approx.)

Energy

Protein

Carbohydrate

Fat

1160

42 g

94 g

65 g

Ingredients :- ☐ Fresh Apricots, halved – 400 gms ☐ Mascarpone cheese – 250 gms ☐ Unsalted Butter – 50 gms ☐ Ginger, – 2" piece ☐ Ginger syrup – 2 tbsp ☐ Lemon Juice – 2 tsp ☐ Sugar – 25 gms ☐ Brandy or liquor – 3 tbsp

Method :- ◊ Finely chop the ginger and mix with the ginger syrup, mascarpone and lemon juice. ◊ Melt the butter in a frying pan and add the sugar. Cook for about 1 minute until the sugar has dissolved.

- Fruits -

Method :- ◊ Add the apricots and fry quickly until lightly coloured but still firm. Stir in the liquor or brandy. ◊ Spoon the mascarpone onto serving plates, top with the fruit and juices. ◊ Serve the dessert warm.

~ ~ ~ ~ ~

- Fruits -

AVOCADO

Avocado is often said to be the most nutritious fruit in the world. It provides more than 25 essential nutrients such as protein, potassium, vitamin E, C, B-vitamins, folic acid, iron, copper, phosphorus and magnesium, just to name a few. It also provides calories for energy and beneficial phytochemicals such as beta-sitosterol, glutathione and lutein.

Avocado contains fat, that is why it is a good source of energy, but the fat in avocado is mostly monounsaturated. In fact, it helps in the absorption of nutrients that are fat-soluble such as alpha and beta-carotene and lutein. It is also high in fiber that is good for the digestive system and the heart. Overall, avocado is considered a complete food. With vitamins, minerals, antioxidants, calories and fiber with no cholesterol and is sodium free.

Avocado is ideal for growing up children, adults and even for babies, especially when blended with other fruits. For athletes, avocado is a nutritious energy booster to rev up the body's strength. It is also a source of linolenic acid (omega-6 fatty acid), which the body converts to gamma-linoleic acid (GLA), a substance that helps to thin the blood, soothe inflammation and improve blood sugar imbalance. It is rich in vitamin E, an antioxidant that detoxifies and boosts resistance to infections. Nutritional Value (100 gms) Calorie 160 Protein 2 g Carbohydrate 8.53 g Fat 14.66 g Fiber 6.7 g

- Fruits -

Avocado's B-vitamin levels help the immune cells to destroy harmful invaders – as does glutathione, a powerful substance that boosts the action of the body's natural killer cells.

Last but not the least, they contain the plant chemical beta-sitosterol which is particularly beneficial to the prostrate gland.

Recipe : Avocado Salsa Nutritional Value (approx.)

Energy

Protein

Carbohydrate

Fat

659

10 g

40 g

60 g

Ingredients :- ☐ Ripe Avocados - 2, small ☐ Spring onions - 8 sticks ☐ Lemon Juice - 2 tbsp ☐ Fresh Coriander, chopped - 2 tbsp ☐ Tomato, finely chopped - 1 ☐ Salt and Pepper - to taste

Method :- ◊ Peel, stone and finely dice avocadoes. ◊ Finely chop and combine with the avocadoes, tomato, lemon juice and coriander leaves. ◊ Season with salt and pepper and serve.

~ ~ ~ ~ ~

- Fruits -

BANANA

In the traditional medicine of India, this golden fruit is regarded as nature's secret of perpetual youth. To this day, banana is known for promoting healthy digestion and creating a feeling of youthfulness. They help promote the retention of calcium, phosphorus and nitrogen - all of which then work to build sound and regenerated tissues. Banana also contains invert sugar, which is an aid to youthful growth and metabolism.

Banana soothes the stomach. Strengthens the stomach lining against acid and ulcers and lab tests show that bananas can act like antibiotics. Very high in potassium, thus may help regulate high blood pressure.

Banana is used as a dietary food against intestinal disorders because of its soft texture and blandness. It is said to contain an unidentified compound called, perhaps jokingly, 'vitamin U' (against ulcer). It is the only raw fruit, which can be eaten without distress in chronic ulcer cases. It neutralizes the over-acidity of the gastric juices and reduces the irritation of the ulcer by coating the lining of the stomach.

Ripe bananas are highly beneficial in the treatment of ulcerative colitis, being bland, smooth, easily-digestible and slightly laxative and they relieve acute symptoms and promote the healing process. Nutritional Value (100 gms) Calorie 89 Protein 1.09 g Carbohydrate 22.84 g Fat 0.33 g Fiber 2.6 g

Bananas are of great value both in constipation and diarrhea as they normalize colonic functions in the large intestine to absorb large amounts of water for proper bowel moments.

Mashed banana together with little salt is a very valuable remedy for dysentery. They are also useful in the treatment of arthritis and gout.

Being high in iron content, bananas are beneficial in the treatment of anaemia. They stimulate the production of haemoglobin in the blood.

The fruit is very useful for those who are allergic to certain foods and who suffer in consequence from skin rashes or digestive disorders or asthma. Unlike other protein foods, many of which contain an amino-acid which these persons cannot tolerate and which causes allergy, bananas contain only benign amino-acids which in most cases are not allergic. The fruit, however, does cause allergic reactions in certain sensitive persons and they should avoid it.

Bananas are valuable in kidney disorder because of their low protein and salt content and high carbohydrate content. They are useful in uremia, a toxic condition of the blood due to kidney congestion and dysfunction. (Those who are suffering from kidney failure because of high blood potassium should not take the fruit.)

Bananas are considered useful in the treatment of tuberculosis; the juice of the plantain or the ordinary cooked bananas works miracles in the cure of tuberculosis.

Juice from Banana stem is a well-known remedy for urinary disorders. It improves the functional efficiency of kidney and liver thereby alleviating the discomforts and diseased condition in them. It clears the excretory organs in the abdominal region of toxins and helps to eliminate them in

the form of urine. It has been found to be of great help in the removal of stones in the kidney, gall bladder, and prostate.

Cooked banana flower eaten with curd is considered an effective medicine for menstrual disorders like painful menstruation and excessive bleeding.

A plaster is prepared by beating a ripe banana into a fine paste. It can be spread over burns and wounds and supported by a cloth bandage. It gives immediate relief. The young tender leaves of banana tree form a cool dressing for inflammations and blisters.

It helps in the recovery from depression and edginess, prevents muscular cramps, improves blood circulation, prevents clot formation and increases heart beat in cases of heart weakness.

Its richness in zinc is helpful in strengthening the hair and prevention of baldness. In external use, it is an effective remedy against warts.

Precautions - Banana, taken as a table fruit, must be thoroughly ripe as otherwise it cannot be digested in the small intestine- which then ferments in the large intestine, often causing wind. Raw bananas contain 20 to 25 per cent starch. But during the process of ripening, this starch is almost wholly converted into assimilable sugar.

Bananas should never be kept in a refrigerator as low temperature prevents their ripening. Those who are suffering from kidney failure because of high blood potassium should not take the fruit.

Recipe : Banana And Walnut Tea Loaf Nutritional Value (approx.)

Energy

Protein

Carbohydrate

Fat

2600

39 g

300 g

149 g

- Fruits -

Ingredients :- ☐ Butter, softened - 100 gms, plus extra for greasing ☐ Sugar 140 gms ☐ Eggs, lightly beaten - 2 ☐ Walnuts - 100 gms ☐ Bananas, mashed - 2 ☐ Milk - 2 tbsp ☐ Self-raising flour - 225 gms

Method :- ◊ Heat oven to 180°C/Gas 4. Grease and line a 900g loaf tin. ◊ Cream the butter and sugar, and then add the eggs. ◊ Set aside 25 g walnuts, then fold the rest into the creamed mixture with the bananas and milk. ◊ Fold in the flour. Spoon into the tin and sprinkle over the reserved walnuts. ◊ Bake for 55 mins-1 hr until risen. Let stand for 10 minutes, then turn out, remove the paper and leave to cool.

~ ~ ~ ~ ~

- Vegetables -

Wonder Food : Vegetables

- Vegetables -

ASPARAGUS

Asparagus is more than just a green vegetable served as a side dish. It's also been recognized historically for its medicinal properties. Down through the ages this popular veggie has been used as a diuretic to reduce water retention and as a laxative due to its high fiber content. Even though you won't find asparagus sold in a drugstore, this popular veggie has some interesting health properties that make it a good addition to almost any diet.

Having an extra order of asparagus may help to protect against unsightly varicose veins. Asparagus is a good source of a flavonoid compound called rutin. Rutin not only has anti-inflammatory properties, but it also helps to improve circulation and strengthen veins and tiny blood vessels known as capillaries – all of which reduce the appearance of varicosities.

Asparagus helps to reduce the risk of heart disease in several ways. It's a good source of potassium to normalize blood pressure, and folate another nutrient important for heart health. It's also rich in soluble fiber to help lower blood cholesterol levels. Asparagus also lowers cholesterol by another mechanism – saponins. Natural saponins found in asparagus bind to cholesterol in the digestive tract so that it's less readily absorbed into the bloodstream. It also alters liver metabolism of cholesterol in a favorable way. All in all, asparagus is one heart friendly vegetable. Nutritional Value (100 gms) Calorie 20 Protein 2.2 g Carbohydrate 3.88 g Fat 0.12 g Fiber 2.1 g

- Vegetables -

Asparagus is a vegetable you can eat without guilt. At twenty-seven calories per cup, it's hard to eat too much of this low calorie veggie. Use it as a side dish instead of potatoes and you'll get more food for fewer calories – and more nutrients too!

Asparagus is an excellent source of folate, a vitamin that's important for reducing the risk of neural tube defects in an unborn baby. Asparagus is a good source of vitamins A and C, antioxidant vitamins that help to protect the skin from free radical damage. Vitamin C is also important for maintaining collagen, a component that gives skin its support structure and prevents sagging.

Asparagus extract may help to prevent hangovers. It seems that asparagus extract boosts enzymes in the liver that break down alcohol. Unfortunately, you'd have to eat the leaves rather than the stalks to get this benefit – or else take an extract.

Asparagus helps in menstrual cramps and is a great food to help treat depression. It has been known to increase the success rate of chemo therapy and helps in getting rid of warts.

The high alkalinity of this wonder juice is effective in reducing the acidity of the blood and helps cleanse the tissues and muscles of waste. A unique phytochemical in asparagus that produces anti-inflammatory effect helps relieve arthritis and rheumatism.

The healthful minerals in asparagus juice make it an important diet for people who are controlling their blood sugar levels. However, it is not to be taken by people with advanced kidney diseases. The diuretic effect of asparagus juice helps relieve premenstrual swelling and bloating. The

- Vegetables -

magnesium in this wonder juice also helps relieve irritability, fatigue, depression, etc.

Caution - Excessive intake of asparagus causes certain uric acid related problems, like gout and kidney stones. Asparagus gives a foul odor to urine.

Recipe : Asparagus Soup Nutritional Value (approx.)

Energy

Protein

Carbohydrate

Fat

772

28.34 g

44.82 g

57.18 g

Ingredients :- □ Butter - 2 tbsp □ Flour - 2 tbsp □ Salt - ½ tsp □ Pepper powder – ¼ tsp □ Milk - 2 cups □ Fresh Asparagus – 400 gms □ Water - enough to boil asparagus

Method :- ◊ To make the white sauce, melt butter in a saucepan over low heat. ◊ Blend in flour, ½ tsp salt and ¼ tsp pepper. ◊ Stir until smooth. Add milk, cook, stirring constantly, until mixture thickens and begins to bubble. ◊ Set aside.

- Vegetables -

Method :- ◊ Wash asparagus and cut in ½ inch pieces. ◊ Cook asparagus in a small amount of boiling water until tender, about 5 minutes. ◊ Drain, reserving the cooking liquid. Set aside a few of the asparagus tips or pieces aside for garnish, if desired. ◊ Mash or blend remaining asparagus; set aside. ◊ Add enough boiling water to cooking liquid to make 1 cup; add white sauce and pureed asparagus. ◊ Heat thoroughly; season to taste with salt and pepper. Add whole asparagus pieces and serve.

~ ~ ~ ~ ~

- Vegetables -

BEETROOT

Beet greens are a very good source of calcium, iron, Vitamins A and C, an excellent source of folic acid, fiber, manganese and potassium. Beet greens and beetroot are a good source of phosphorus, magnesium, iron and vitamin B6. Betacyanin is the pigment that gives beetroot its color, and has powerful antioxidant properties.

Beet fiber has been shown to have cholesterol lowering capabilities.

Beetroot juice has been shown to lower blood pressure in subjects with normal blood pressure. Betaine, a nutrient found in beets lowers plasma homocysteine, a possible risk factor for cardiovascular disease and also supports healthy liver function. When the liver is functioning properly, fats are broken down efficiently, aiding weight loss, and preventing fatigue and nausea.

Preliminary tests suggest that beetroot ingestion can be one of the useful means to prevent lung and skin cancer. Other studies have shown that beet juice inhibits the formation of cancer causing compounds called nitrosamines. Folate, nitrates, magnesium and antioxidants in beet juice, beet fiber and beet greens have been shown to aid in disease prevention and control as well as colon and stomach cancer prevention. The red pigment in beets raises antioxidant enzyme levels in the liver and may promote detoxification in the intestines, blood and liver. Colon cancer Nutritional Value (100 gms) Calorie 43 Protein 1.61 g Carbohydrate 9.56 g Fat 0.17 g Fiber 2.8 g

- Vegetables -

research has also shown that consumption of beet fiber may increase colonic CD8 cells, which detect and remove abnormal cells.

Beet juice also inhibits the production of nitrosamines from foods containing nitrates in stomach cancer patients. For beets to be most useful in cancer prevention they should be taken uncooked or very lightly cooked as heat reduces their anti-cancer properties. Folate is considered an important aid in maintaining a healthy pregnancy. It is critical at times of rapid cell development as it is necessary for creating DNA and RNA. The high level of folate (up to 136 grams per cup) in beets makes them a valuable food for pregnancy. Spina bifida and anencephaly are two birth defects which may be prevented by the consumption of folate rich foods.

Magnesium is an important mineral in healthy bone production and maintenance. Without appropriate levels of magnesium, calcium cannot be utilized effectively. Beet root is high in magnesium, making it a good vegetable for women concerned with preventing osteoporosis. A word of caution; beet greens are high in oxalic acid which interferes with calcium metabolism, so the greens should not be consumed in any significant quantities by osteoporosis sufferers.

Alzheimer's disease and senile dementia are two types of cognitive disorders. Antioxidants have been shown to be useful in the prevention of these cognitive problems. Dark skinned vegetables such as beets are high in those antioxidants known to lower the levels of free radicals in the body which are, in part, responsible for cell damage in the brain as well as other parts of the body. While all of this information about the value of beets may lead some to consider it to be the next new superfood, it is important to keep some perspective. Many other fresh fruits and

- Vegetables -

vegetables have similar properties so it makes sense to include a variety of these foods in the diet to maintain optimum health.

Beets are of great therapeutic value. They have properties to clean the kidneys and gall bladder. Being rich in alkaline elements, potassium, calcium, magnesium and iron, they are useful in combating acidosis and aid the natural processes of elimination. Red beet juice is associated with human blood and blood forming qualities. Due to its higher content of iron, it regenerates and reactivates the red blood cells, supplies fresh oxygen to the body and helps the normal function of vesicular breathing i.e. normal breath sound. It is thus extremely useful in the treatment of anaemia.

Beet juice is beneficial in the treatment of jaundice, hepatitis, nausea and vomiting due to biliousness, diarrhoea and dysentery. Adding a teaspoonful of lime juice to this juice increases its medicinal value and can be given as a liquid food in these conditions. Fresh beet juice mixed with a tablespoonful of honey taken every morning before breakfast helps the healing of gastric ulcer.

Leaves of beet root, eaten as green-leafy vegetable and its juice, mixed with lime juice, are also valuable in jaundice and gastric ulcer. The juice should be taken once daily. The cellulose content of the beet acts as a bulk residue, increases peristalsis. Its regular use thus prevents habitual constipation. A decoction of the beet root is highly valuable in chronic constipation and haemorrhoids, i.e. piles.

The beet juice is an excellent solvent for inorganic calcium deposits. It is, therefore, valuable in the treatment of hypertension, arteriosclerosis, heart trouble and varicose veins. The beet juice, in combination with the juice of carrot and cucumber, is one of the finest cleansing material for

- Vegetables -

kidneys and gall bladder. It is highly beneficial in all disorders relating to these two organs.

The water in which beet roots and tops have been boiled is an excellent application for boils, skin inflammation and outbreaks of pimples and pustules. The white beet is better for this purpose. For an irritable skin the body should be sponged down occasionally with a mixture of three parts of beet water to one part of white vinegar. This mixture is also useful as a skin wash in cases of measles and eruptive fevers. The decoction of beets mixed with little vinegar can be used externally to cleanse scurf or dandruff from the head. For dandruff, the beet water should also be massaged into the scalp with the ginger tip every night.

Recipe : Hot Beet Soup Nutritional Value (approx.)

Energy

Protein

Carbohydrate

Fat

336

8 g

49 g

15 g

Ingredients :- ☐ Onion, peeled, chopped - 1 ☐ Garlic, crushed - 1 clove ☐ Chili Powder - 1 tsp ☐ Olive oil - 1 tbsp ☐ Tomatoes - 400 gms ☐ Beetroot - 2 ☐ Sour cream - to serve

- Vegetables -

Method :- ◊ Preheat the oven to 200°C / 400°F / gas mark 6 ◊ Wrap each beetroot in foil and bake for about 45 minutes until tender. ◊ Leave them to cool and then peel and dice. ◊ Sauté the garlic and onions over a low heat in the olive oil for 3 minutes. ◊ Add the chili powder, stir together for a minute. ◊ Add tomatoes and bring to the boil. ◊ Simmer for 15 minutes before stirring in the beetroot. ◊ Pour the soup into bowls, add some sour cream and serve.

~ ~ ~ ~ ~

- Vegetables -

BITTER GOURD

Bitter Gourd, also known as balsam apple, bitter-melon and balsam pear, is renowned in the Old World tropics for its medicinal properties. From India to the Federated States of Micronesia, and from China to the Solomon Islands, this bitter fruit is part of medicinal folklore as well as an exotic, acquired taste.

The New World is slowly beginning to discover for itself the ability of this versatile fruit to treat diseases as old as diabetes and as new as HIV/AIDS.

Bitter gourds are very low in calories but dense with precious nutrients. It is an excellent source of vitamins B1, B2, and B3, C, magnesium, folic acid, zinc, phosphorus, manganese, and has high dietary fiber. It is rich in iron, contains twice the beta-carotene of broccoli, twice the calcium of spinach and twice the potassium of a banana.

Bitter gourd juice is highly beneficial for treating blood disorders like blood boils and itching due to toxemia.

Bitter melon contains a hypoglycemic compound (a plant insulin) that is highly beneficial in lowering sugar levels in blood and urine. Bitter melon juice has been shown to significantly improve glucose tolerance without increasing blood insulin levels. Nutritional Value (100 gms) Calorie 17 Protein 1 g Carbohydrate 3.7 g Fat 0.2 g Fiber 2.8 g

- Vegetables -

Regular consumption of bitter gourd juice has been proven to improve energy and stamina level. Even sleeping patterns have been shown to have improved/stabilized.

The high beta-carotene and other properties in bitter gourd make it one of the finest vegetable-fruit that help alleviate eye problems and improving eyesight. Bitter melon juice may be beneficial in the treatment of a hangover for its alcohol intoxication properties. It also helps to cleanse and repair and nourish liver problems due to alcohol consumption.

This bitter juice can also help to build your immune system and increase your body's resistance against infection. To hasten healing, use the paste of the roots of bitter melon plant and apply over the piles.

Regular consumption of this bitter juice has also been known to improve psoriasis condition and other fungal infections like ring-worm and athlete's feet. Drink it daily to improve asthma, bronchitis and pharyngitis.

Bitter gourd contains beneficial properties that cleanse the blood of toxins. It is also helpful in getting rid of jaundice for the same reasons.

The bitter gourd has excellent medicinal virtues. It is antidotal, antipyretic tonic, appetizing, stomachic, antibilious and laxative.

The seeds became a cure-all of sorts, finding their way into remedies for conditions as different and unrelated to each other as mumps, lumbago (low back pain), breast cancer and piles. Juice from crushed leaves was a liver tonic and menstrual regulator; crushed flowers and roots were cough remedies and asthma fix-its.

- Vegetables -

Bitter gourd is a blood purifier, activates spleen and liver and is highly beneficial in diabetes. It is a purgative, appetizer, digestive, anti-inflammatory and has healing capacity.

With the juice of bitter gourd you can massage the affected portion and also eat bitter gourd to cure joint pains.

Daily intake of a tea spoon of bitter gourd juice, continued for a few days, destroys stomach worms.

Recipe : Stuffed Bitter Gourd Nutritional Value (approx.)

Energy

Protein

Carbohydrate

Fat

368

39 g

50 g

4 g

Ingredients :- ☐ Bitter Gourd(Peeled , washed deseeded and deep fried) - 5 ☐ Paneer- 250 gms ☐ Onion - 1 medium ☐ Tomato - 1 medium ☐ Salt to taste ☐ Oil for deep frying ☐ Red Chili powder – to taste ☐ Turmeric powder - ¼ tsp ☐ Coriander leaves – 1 tbsp ☐ Garam Masala - ½ tsp

- Vegetables -

Method :- ◊ Crumble the paneer & add to it the spices (salt & red pepper) ◊ Now fill the gourds with this paneer. ◊ Take little oil in Karahi (wok) & fry chopped onions till transparent. ◊ Now add chopped tomatoes & fry for just a minute. ◊ Add the dry spices in the tomatoes (salt, pepper, turmeric). ◊ Add the stuffed gourd to the Karahi & mix well ◊ Make sure the stuffing doesn't come out. If there is little paneer left put it in along with gourd. ◊ Let it be on medium flame for 10 minutes. Fold in occasionally. ◊ Now add chopped coriander & Garam masala & serve hot as a side dish with Roti / Rice.

~ ~ ~ ~ ~

- Vegetables -

BOTTLE GOURD

Bottle gourd is one of the favorite vegetable of Indians and has numerous health benefits. They are especially good for aged people.

The cooked vegetable is cooling, diuretic, sedative and anti bilious. It gives a feeling of relaxation after eating. However, bottle gourd should not be eaten in a raw state as it may prove harmful for stomach and intestines.

Bottle gourd is very valuable in urinary disorders. It serves as an alkaline mixture. It should be given with sulpha drugs in the treatment of urinal infection. It acts as an alkaline diuretic in this condition.

The juice of bottle gourd is a valuable medicine for excessive thirst due to severe diarrhea, diabetes and excessive use of fatty or fried foods. Its use during summer prevents excessive loss of sodium, quenches thirst and helps in preventing fatigue.

The mixture of bottle gourd juice and sesame oil acts as an effective medicine for insomnia. It should be massaged over scalp every night. The cooked leaves of bottle gourd are also beneficial in the treatment of insomnia.

Cooked bottle gourd is cooling, calming, diuretic and easy to digest. It is also effective against constipation and other digestive disorders. It carries the potential for breaking calculus (stones) in body. This vegetable is very good for balancing liver function. It is often recommended by ayurvedic Nutritional Value (100 gms) Calorie 12 Protein 0.2 g Carbohydrate 2.5 g Fat 0.1 g Fiber 0.6 g

- Vegetables -

physicians when the liver is inflamed and cannot efficiently process food for maximum nutrition and assimilation.

Drink bottle gourd juice once daily early in the morning for treating graying hair. The juice is useful in treating insanity, epilepsy & other nervous diseases.

Recently, bottle gourd has attracted a lot of attention due to its importance in treatment of blood pressure and heart disease.

The pulp around the seed is emetic and purgative. A poultice of the crushed leaves should be applied to the head to treat headaches. The flowers are an antidote to poison. The stem, bark and the rind of the fruit are diuretic. The fruit is antilithic, diuretic, emetic and refrigerant.

Recipe : Bottle Gourd Chutney Nutritional Value (approx.)

Energy

Protein

Carbohydrate

Fat

195

25 g

35 g

7 g

Ingredients :- ☐ Bottle gourd - 1/2 ☐ Garlic - 3 cloves ☐ Red chili, dry - 3 (Depends on your spice tolerance) ☐ Tomato, ripen - 1 ☐ Coriander leaves - 3 to 4 sprigs ☐ Salt - to taste ☐ Oil – 1 tsp For tempering: ☐ Mustard seeds and Urad dal - ½ tsp each ☐ Curry leaves - a sprig

- Vegetables -

Method :- ◊ Remove the skin of bottle gourd and cut it into pieces. ◊ Cut tomato into pieces. ◊ Crush the garlic cloves and remove the skin. Keep all this aside. ◊ Heat oil in a pan. Add red chilies and crushed garlic cloves, fry till garlic turns into golden brown. ◊ Add bottle gourd pieces and fry for 3 to 5 minutes. ◊ Add Tomato pieces and fry again for 3 to 5 minutes. ◊ Finally add coriander leaves, curry leaves and salt. Remove from heat. ◊ Once it cools off, grind this in a blender or in a food processor. ◊ Transfer it to a serving bowl. ◊ For the tempering: heat a teaspoon of oil in a pan. Add Mustard seeds and Urad dal. Once it splutters, add curry leaves and fry for 30 seconds. Pour this mix to the ground chutney.

~ ~ ~ ~ ~

- Pulses -

Wonder Food : Pulses

- Pulses -

BENGAL GRAM

Bengal gram is one of the most important pulses in India. It is consumed in the form of whole dried seeds and in the form of dhal, prepared by splitting the seeds in a mill and separating the husk. Seeds are angular with pointed beak and small hilum. All parts of the plant are covered with glandular hairs.

Soaked in water overnight and chewed in the morning with honey, the whole gram seed acts as a general tonic. The liquid, obtained by soaking the seeds and then macerating them, also serves as tonic. Sprouted Bengal grams supply plenty of B-complex and vitamins.

Cooked germinated gram is a wholesome food for children and invalids. However excessive use of Bengal gram causes indigestion and may precipitate urinary calcium due to high concentration of oxalic acid and form urinary stone of calculi.

Experiments have shown that the intake of water extract of Bengal gram enhances the utilization of glucose in both the diabetic and normal persons. Liberal usage of Bengal gram extracts, have shown considerable improvement in fasting blood sugar levels, glucose tolerance, urinary excretion of sugar and general health.

Fresh juice of Bengal gram leaves is a very rich source of iron. It is therefore, highly beneficial in the treatment of iron deficiency and anaemia. Nutritional Value (100 gms) Calorie 360 Protein 17.1 g Carbohydrate 60.9 g Fat 5.3 g Fiber 3.9 g

- Pulses -

An acidic liquid is obtained by collecting the dew drops from the leaves by spreading a thin white cloth over the crop at night or by any other means. This acidic liquid contains about 94 per cent malic acid and 6 per cent oxalic acid and is used medicinally. It is a valuable astringent useful in dyspepsia, vomiting, indigestion, costiveness, diarrhea and dysentery.

A bath prepared by putting an entire Bengal gram plant in hot water is highly beneficial in painful menstruation. It may be taken in the form of a sitting steam bath.

Bengal gram flour is a very effective cleansing agent and its regular use as a cosmetic bleaches the skin. In allergic skin diseases like eczema, contact dermatitis, scabies, washing the skin with this flour will be highly beneficial. The Bengal gram flour can be beneficially used in the treatment of pimples.

Washing hair with Bengal gram flour keeps them clean, soft and free from hair diseases. Flour of the puffed Bengal gram is a very nutritive food and an effective remedy for impotency and premature ejaculation. For better results, two tablespoonful of this flour should be mixed with sugar, powdered dates and skimmed milk powder. It can be packed in airtight tins and used when required.

Recipe : Chana Dal Rice Nutritional Value (approx.) (approx.)

Energy

Protein

Carbohydrate

Fat

1175

38 g

139 g

58 g

- Pulses -

Ingredients :- ☐ Rice - 1 cup ☐ Chana Dal - ½ cup ☐ Peanuts - 1 tsp ☐ Oil - 3 tbsp ☐ Garlic, chopped - 1 tbsp ☐ Ginger, chopped - 2 tbsp ☐ Salt - to taste ☐ Onion, chopped - 1 ☐ Water - 2 cups ☐ Mustard seeds - 1 tsp ☐ Black Pepper powder - 3 tsp ☐ Curry leaves - 6

Method :- ◊ Wash chana dal and soak for 5-6 hours. ◊ Wash rice and soak for 1 hour. ◊ Heat oil in a pan. Add mustard seeds and let them crackle. ◊ Add garlic, ginger and onion and sauté till the onions turn light brown. ◊ Add the chana dal, curry leaves and 2 tbsp water. Sauté it for 2 minutes. ◊ Add the rice with two cups of water and salt. ◊ Add black pepper when it starts boiling. ◊ Cover and cook on medium flame till done, stirring at regular intervals.

- Pulses -

Method :- ◊ Serve hot, garnish with chopped coriander leaves.

~ ~ ~ ~ ~

- Pulses -

BLACK-EYED BEAN

Not only Black-eyed beans are low in fat and high in quality protein, but they also have the added bonus of soluble fiber's disease-preventing qualities. The soluble fiber in beans dissolves in water, trapping bile acids in its gummy goo. This lowers blood levels of damaging LDL cholesterol, especially if LDL cholesterol levels were high to begin with, without compromising the level of protective HDL cholesterol.

Because beans are singled out for their soluble fiber, you may not realize they also provide substantial insoluble fiber, which helps combat constipation, colon cancer, and other conditions that afflict your digestive tract.

Insoluble fiber absorbs water, which swells the size of stool, puts pressure on the intestines, and moves everything along faster. To help combat the gas problem -- caused by indigestible carbohydrates -- let your body get used to eating beans. Start slowly, eating only small amounts at first, and try to eat them when you know you'll be active afterward; it helps break up the gas.

Black-eye peas contain several types of phytochemicals. They are rich in lignans, which may play a role in preventing osteoporosis, heart disease, and certain cancers. The flavonoids in beans may help reduce heart disease and cancer risk. Phytosterols, also found in legumes, help reduce Nutritional Value (100 gms) Calorie 341 Protein 21.6 g Carbohydrate 62.3 g Fat 1.42 g Fiber 15.2 g

- Pulses -

blood cholesterol levels. Black-eyed peas provide a number of nutrients, are a rich source of fiber and can be used in a number of recipes. For vegetarians, such beans can provide a needed source of iron. No matter how you choose to prepare them, black-eyed peas can be a wonderful supplement to your healthy eating plan. The common commercial one is called the California Blackeye; it is pale-colored with a prominent black spot.

Recipe : Black-Eyed Bean Rice Nutritional Value (approx.)

Energy

Protein

Carbohydrate

Fat

769

37 g

134 g

13 g

Ingredients :- ☐ Black-Eyed Bean, cooked - 350 gms ☐ Basmati rice, cooked - 150 gms ☐ Spring onions, chopped - 5 ☐ Olive oil - 2 tsp ☐ Water - 2 tbsp ☐ Juice of 1 lemon ☐ Chili powder - ½ tsp ☐ Cumin seeds - ½ tsp ☐ Fresh Coriander, chopped - 2 tbsp ☐ Salt, pepper - to taste

Method :- ◊ Gently fry the onions in the oil until golden. ◊ Add all the remaining ingredients, apart from the rice, stir and

- Pulses -

Method :- heat through for 2 minutes. ◊ Add the rice and pepper and stir-fry for a further 2 minutes. ◊ Serve hot.

~ ~ ~ ~ ~

- Cereal s -

Wonder Food : Cereals

- Cereal s -

BROWN RICE

Brown rice is an excellent source of magnesium, iron, selenium, manganese, and the vitamins B1, B2, B3, and B6. Brown rice is a good source of dietary fiber, protein, and gamma-oryzanol. White rice is brown rice that has had essential nutrients removed when processed in order to make it easier and faster to cook, and to give it a longer shelf life. This is accomplished by removing the bran, and with it, minerals and vitamins that are necessary in our diet.

Inositol hexaphosphate, a naturally occurring molecule found in high-fiber foods such as brown rice, is a compound that has been shown to demonstrate cancer prevention properties. Inositol hexaphosphate holds great promise in strategies for the prevention and treatment of cancer.

Pancreatic cancer is an extremely virulent form of cancer with few effective treatments. An in vitro study has suggested that inositol hexaphosphate may be a therapy for treatment of pancreatic cancer.

Brown rice has a rich content of manganese, which helps in the production of energy from carbohydrates and protein. The nutrient also plays a key role in the synthesis of fatty acids, which is necessary for a Nutritional Value (100 gms) Calorie 362 Protein 7.5 g Carbohydrate 76.17 g Fat 2.68 g Fiber 3.4 g

- Cereal s -

healthy nervous system. One can get about 88% of the daily need of manganese by consuming just one cup of brown rice.

The manganese present in brown rice is also required for the antioxidant enzyme, super oxide dismutase, which protects the mitochondria against the free radicals formed during energy production.

Brown rice is a rich source of fiber and selenium, both of which help lower the risk of colon cancer significantly. Selenium also works with vitamin E, in several antioxidant systems of the body, which help fight against heart diseases. This is also beneficial against the symptoms of asthma and rheumatoid arthritis.

The rice also contains insoluble fiber, which helps women avoid developing gallstones. It is rich in fiber, which contributes towards the reduction of cholesterol level and also the prevention of atherosclerosis. The fiber also binds to the cancer-causing chemicals, protecting the body against colon cancer. The fiber present in brown rice also helps normalize the bowel function and thus, reduces constipation.

The oil present in brown rice helps in lowering the cholesterol level in the body. Brown rice is extremely good for postmenopausal women with complains of high blood pressure, high cholesterol, and other symptoms of cardiovascular diseases.

It contains phytonutrients, which are highly beneficial for sound health.

Brown rice is abundant in plant lignans, which get converted into mammalian lignans like enterolactone, in the intestine. Enterolactone is highly protective against breast and other hormone-dependent cancers and also heart diseases.

- Cereal s -

The rice helps in reducing the risk of insulin resistance and the metabolic syndrome. Metabolic syndrome is associated with symptoms like visceral obesity, high triglycerides, high blood pressure and low level of defensive HDL cholesterol.

Brown rice reduces the risk of type 2 diabetes. Brown rice is a good source of magnesium, which reduces the severity of asthma, lowers the frequency of migraine headaches and decreases the risk of heart attack and stroke. Magnesium balances the action of calcium and thus, helps in regulating nerve and muscle tone.

Brown rice offers major protection against breast cancer, especially in pre-menopausal women. Intake of brown rice can help the body fight against childhood asthma. It is also protective against obesity, ischemic stroke and insulin resistance.

Caution - Brown rice is not seen to have any negative effect on the body, including any allergic effect. It does not contain any significant amount of oxalates and purines. However, the rice that is not grown organically is seen to contain traces of arsenic. Though low doses of arsenic are not seen to cause any serious diseases, its heavy intake can make one more susceptible to the risk of cancer. So, always go for the organically grown brown rice, as it is free of arsenic content.

Recipe : Brown Rice Pudding With Sultanas And Almonds Nutritional Value (approx.)

Energy

Protein

Carbohydrate

Fat

860

100 g

135 g

30 g

- Cereal s -

Ingredients :- ☐ Brown Rice – 75 gms ☐ Milk – 900 ml ☐ Sugar – 25 gms ☐ Sultanas – 75 gms ☐ Grated nutmeg – ½ tsp ☐ Butter – 15 gms ☐ Ginger – ½ inch ☐ Flaked almonds – to garnish

Method :- ◊ Wash the rice and cook for 15 minutes. ◊ Drain the water and again boil it with milk and the sugar. ◊ Pour into a buttered oven proof dish. ◊ Add the sultanas and stir. ◊ Sprinkle over the nutmeg and dot with butter. ◊ Cook in the oven, at 180 degree Celsius for 1 ½ -2 hours, stirring twice. ◊ Sprinkle with chopped ginger and flaked almonds. ◊ Serve.

~ ~ ~ ~ ~

- Dry Fruit s -

Wonder Food : Dry Fruits

- Dry Fruit s -

ALMOND

Chewing a few almonds seems to relieve heartburn because of their high oil content. Eating almonds is supposed to lower the risk of cancer and to lower cholesterol. The high calcium level of almonds may lower the risk of colon and rectal cancers. The high levels of antioxidant flavonoids in the almond skin help to inhibit the oxidation of low density lipoproteins, thereby reducing the formation of plaques in the arteries. The extracted oil, which is edible and has a nutty taste, is used to clear the skin of spots.

Both the sweet and bitter varieties of almonds have quite a few medicinal qualities when used in the right way. Sweet almonds are very high in protein. Both types of almonds reduce inflammation and are used in the treatment of bronchitis. In addition to being an excellent source of protein, as mentioned above, almonds are also a source of healthy fat, zinc, potassium, iron, B vitamins, and magnesium.

Almonds are also known to aid respiration, act as a digestive aid and even can help with urinary problems.

The medicinal virtues of almonds help the formation of new blood cells, haemoglobin and play a major role in maintaining the smooth physiological functions of brain, nerves, bones, heart and liver. The almond is thus highly beneficial in preserving the vitality of the brain, in Nutritional Value (100 gms) Calorie 575 Protein 21.22 g Carbohydrate 21.67 g Fat 49.42 g Fiber 12.2 g strengthening the muscles and in prolonging life. It forms a vital part of all tonic preparation in Ayurveda and Unani Medicines.

Paste of almond with milk, cream and fresh rose bud's paste prevents early appearance of wrinkles, black heads, dryness of the skin, pimples and keeps the face fresh. A teaspoonful of almond oil mixed with a teaspoonful of amla juice, massaged over scalp, is a valuable remedy for falling hair, thinness of hair, dandruff and premature graying of hair.

Almonds should be consumed properly for beneficial results. The skin of almonds should always be removed before use as it contains irritating properties. This can be done by soaking them in water for one or two hours.

Almonds contain copper in organic form at the rate of 1.15 mg per 100 grams. The copper along with iron and vitamins acts as a catalyst in the synthesis of blood haemoglobin. Almonds are therefore, a useful food remedy for anaemia.

The use of almonds has proved highly beneficial for the treatment of chronic constipation. It is an excellent laxative. 11 to 15 kernels taken at bed time will facilitate a clear motion the next morning. Those who suffer from weak stomach can take seven grams of almond oil with hot milk.

Wild almonds are considered useful in skin diseases, especially eczema. In case of inflammatory condition of the skin, the external application of almond oil will ease the pain and cool the heat.

An emulsion of almonds is useful in bronchial diseases, hoarseness and tickling cough and is also useful in whooping cough, bronchitis and asthma.

Almonds are very useful in case of loss of sexual energy which usually results from nervous debility and brain weakness. Their regular use will strengthen sexual power. Chewing of equal quantity of almond kernels and roasted gram also helps in restoring sexual vigor.

Recipe : Cherry Almond Loaf Nutritional Value (approx.)

Energy

Protein

Carbohydrate

Fat

3353.5

60.17 g

346.17 g

200.5 g

Ingredients :- ☐ Refined Flour - 1 cup ☐ Oil - ½ cup ☐ Powdered sugar - 3/4 cup ☐ Eggs - 4 ☐ Baking Powder - 2 tsp ☐ Glazed Cherries - 1 cup ☐ Almonds, chopped roughly - 100 gms ☐ Vanilla essence - 3 drops

Method :- ◊ Grease and dust a baking tin. ◊ Pre heat the oven at 150°C, 300°F. ◊ Sieve the flour and baking powder 2-3 times and keep aside. ◊ Keeping aside a few cherries and almond for garnishing, lightly mix the rest of them with the sieved flour. ◊ Beat sugar and eggs in a pan till frothy.

- Dry Fruit s -

Method :- ◊ Add oil gradually and keep beating all the time. ◊ Add the flour to the batter. Beat well. ◊ Add essence and mix well. ◊ The batter should be quite thick but it should be such that it can be spooned out. ◊ Put the batter in the prepared tin. Sprinkle the chopped fruits on top. ◊ Bake in the oven for an hour. ◊ Pancake is done. Remove from the oven. ◊ Let it cool for 10 minutes and then remove the tin. ◊ Serve warm.

~ ~ ~ ~ ~

-

www.ingramcontent.com/pod-product-compliance
Lightning Source LLC
Chambersburg PA
CBHW071152280526
45787CB00003B/1497